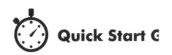 **Quick Start G**

The Essential
800 CALORIE
MEDITERRANEAN
Recipe Book

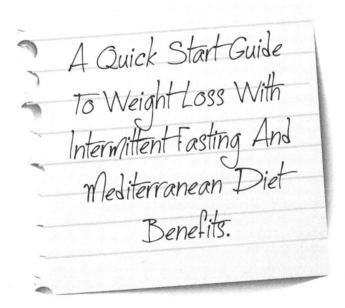

A Quick Start Guide To Weight Loss With Intermittent Fasting And Mediterranean Diet Benefits.

Calorie Counted Low Carb Healthy Recipes.

REVISED EDITION

First published in 2019 by Erin Rose Publishing

Text and illustration copyright © 2019 Erin Rose Publishing

Design: Julie Anson

ISBN: 978-1-9161523-0-4

A CIP record for this book is available from the British Library.

DISCLAIMER: This book is for informational purposes only and not intended as a substitute for the medical advice, diagnosis or treatment of a physician or qualified healthcare provider. The reader should consult a physician before undertaking a new health care regime and in all matters relating to his/her health, and particularly with respect to any symptoms that may require diagnosis or medical attention.

While every care has been taken in compiling the recipes for this Book we cannot accept responsibility for any problems which arise as a result of preparing one of the recipes. The author and publisher disclaim responsibility for any adverse effects that may arise from the use or application of the recipes in this book. Some of the recipes in this book include nuts. If you have a nut allergy it's important to avoid these.

CONTENTS

Breakfast, Lunch & Dinner

Recipes Under 100 Calories

Recipes Under 200 Calories

Recipes Under 300 Calories

Recipes Under 400 Calories

Recipes Under 500 Calories

Desserts Under 230 Calories

INTRODUCTION

Bringing together the world's most successful diets, this easy-to-use cookbook provides you with simple and delicious recipes for fast, healthy weight loss.

By combining intermittent fasting (IF) with easy, healthy and delicious low carb, calorie-counted, Mediterranean style recipes, you can maximise weight loss.

You can tailor your diet depending on your life-style and how much weight you want to lose. This book guides you on how to get started, offering weight loss tips and plenty of lovely recipes to choose from.

The Mediterranean Diet has been repeatedly backed by science which proved the health benefits include improving longevity, helping reduce cholesterol levels, blood pressure, heart disease, strokes, blood sugar levels, diabetes, obesity and inflammation.

Intermittent fasting on the 5:2 diet has been a great success with thousands achieving and maintaining their weight loss goals by significantly restricting their calorie intake 2 days a week. New research shows the optimum number of calories you can consume and still lose weight is 800 calories per day which is much more doable. Team that with the health benefits of the Mediterranean style food and you have a winner!

This **Quick Start Guide** contains clear, concise information on achieving fast weight loss and sustainable health benefits. It provides you with the essential information, plus, simple, great-tasting, calorie-counted recipes which are also low in carbohydrates. The result - you will be able to prevent hunger while losing weight and improving your health!

800 Calories For Optimum Weight Loss

A Newcastle University published results of a study which found that overweight, type 2 diabetics who followed an 800-calorie-a-day diet for 12 weeks 'reversed' their diabetes, plus they achieved and sustained average weight loss of 10kg.

A study by Oxford University showed health markers, including an improvement in metabolic and cardiovascular health, plus an average 10kg weight loss in an overweight group who replaced meals with soups, shakes and bars which totalled 800 calories per day.

A daily limit of 800 calories is about a third of the average guidelines to maintain weight, which for a man is 2,500 calories and less than half that recommended for a woman, which is 2,000 calories.

Simply put, the 800 calorie diet plan involves restricting calories, on a daily basis, for no more than 12 weeks. Or following the 5:2 diet plan by consuming up to 800 calories 2 days a week, whilst eating a normal healthy diet for the 5 days.

Such calorie restriction is safe and doable for most people. Contrary to belief, fast weight loss can be maintained and it can help to lower blood sugar levels, in some cases even reversing pre-diabetes and type 2 diabetes.

By restricting calories you will be reducing, or cutting out, junk food, including refined carbohydrates, sugars and harmful fats on fasting days. Instead you will be eating vegetables, healthy fats and quality protein. This will have beneficial changes on the health of your gut too.

Eating low carbohydrate foods improves blood sugar, reduces your waistline and boosts your health. Blood sugar rises every time we eat, even more so from rapidly absorbed sugars and starchy carbohydrates. It later falls, when the quick effect of the quickly absorbed food wears off, causing peaks and troughs in the blood sugar causing hunger, fatigue and cravings for more sugar. To prevent huge swings in your blood sugar it is best to avoid starchy carbohydrates, sugar and alcohol to stabilise the body.

Another popular and proven successful weight loss technique is Time Restricted Eating (TRE). Basically this means eating all calories within a certain time frame each day. Often this can be a window of 8 to 16 hours a day, stretching the overnight fasting period, so you would consume no calories during this time. Time restricted eating allows the body to repair and you can start with a shorter fasting time and gradually increase it.

The benefits of calorie restriction and intermittent fasting extend beyond weight loss, and it is suitable for most people who are overweight. However, check with your doctor or health care professional that it is safe for you to do so before you begin.

> **Fasting is not suitable for the elderly, convalescing, children, during pregnancy or breastfeeding, or if you suffer from or have a history of an eating disorder or have a low BMI or have other medical conditions. Always seek your doctor's advice and especially regarding medication changes.**

How to Get Started

Beginning any diet can be daunting so allow yourself to do it in whatever way works best for you. Of course, this all depends on how much weight you want to lose and how quickly you want to shed the extra pounds.

You can:

1. **Restrict yourself to 800 calories a day for a minimum of 2 weeks and up to a maximum of 12 weeks.**

2. **Follow the 5:2 diet, restricting yourself to 800 calories for 2 days a week and eating sensibly for 5 days.**

3. **Combine fasting and/or non-fasting days with time restricted eating. This means all food should be eaten in an 8–12 hour window each day.**

Plan which days you are fasting so you can be prepared. Increase your fluid intake on these days. Not only will it replace your usual food intake it will help your body eliminate fat. Drinking 2-3 litres a day is advisable.

Avoiding processed foods, sugar and carbohydrates such as pasta, bread, biscuits, cakes, cereals, crackers, noodles, rice and potatoes. Beware of sugary sauces like sweet chilli, BBQ, ketchup and concentrated fruit juices or fast food containing hidden sugars. Processed food are often contain high amounts of sugar and fat and it's thought that combination is what causes cravings for junk food and results in weight gain.

Familiarise yourself with what you can eat and remove tempting foods from your cupboards.

You can eat your daily calorie limit over 2 or 3 meals, depending on what suits you and fits in with your lifestyle. Some prefer to extend their overnight fasting by having a late breakfast and early evening meal as they find it easier. However, you can spread your calorie intake over breakfast, lunch and dinner, opting for lighter meals.

This may take a little experimenting and adapting as you begin your diet and work out what works best for you.

You can choose to stick to 800 calories a day for 14 days, or however long you decide, depending on how rapidly you want to lose weight and then switch to the 5:2 diet. Eating low carbohydrate foods will reduce any cravings or hunger pangs making it much easier for you. Eating protein will help you feel satiated for longer.

The recipes are all calorie counted and listed according to their calorie content. This will make it easy to select what to have for each meal. You can choose whether to have 2 or 3 meals a day. The recipes can be used for whichever meal you choose – just stay within the 800 calorie total on fasting days.

This cookbook also contains recipes for healthy, low-carb, low-calorie desserts, however only eat these in moderation and avoid them completely if you have sugar cravings. These can be reduced or eliminated completely by avoiding sugar and starchy carbohydrates.

Diet Tips

- Staying busy will help take your mind of food, especially when you first start. Get up and do something. Exercise helps, even if it's going for a walk.

- Keep a food diary. Writing down what you eat helps you track your calorie consumption and you can also log how you are feeling including energy, sleep, weight loss and fluid intake. It's great to reflect and see how you're doing.

- Decide when the best time to fast is. Avoiding social get-togethers, holidays and weekends will help you kick start your plan.

- On non-fasting days, don't binge. You can stick to the low carb recipes and don't over-do the portions.

- Avoid refined carbohydrates and sugars and eat vegetables and protein.

- You can fill up on high volume foods like broccoli, cauliflower, carrots and heaps of lettuce or spinach without adding large amounts of calories.

- At mealtimes, replace starchy carbohydrates with lots of veggies and you'll feel less sluggish and hungry.

- Schedule in easy meals, plan in advance so you avoid temptation. That way you can also avoid missing a meal.

- Drink plenty of water!

- If you get sugar cravings, they will pass! Once your body switches to burning fat for fuel it will be easier.

- You may experience headaches in the first couple of days as your body adjusts. Relax, relax and drink water. Remember, you need extra fluid as your body burns off fat.

- Prepare some tasty meals and snacks for the fridge or freezer and plan ahead so you aren't tempted to overdo the calories.

- Finding a diet buddy is not only god for moral but you can also swap ideas, recipes and provide encouragement.

- Experiment. You're bound to find your own staples which are handy and quick to prepare.

BREAKFAST, LUNCH & DINNER

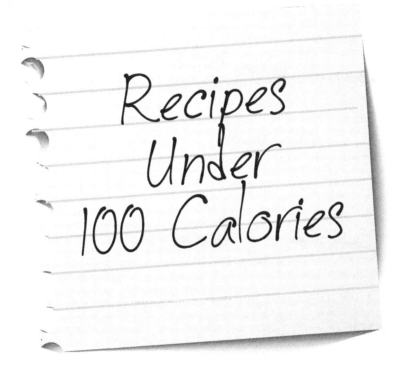

Recipes Under 100 Calories

Creamy Red Pepper Soup

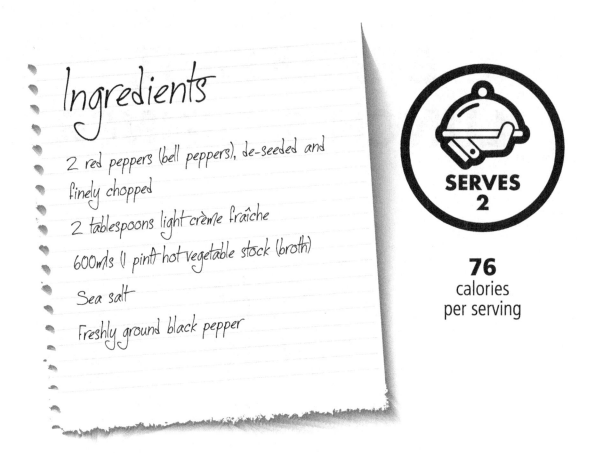

Ingredients

2 red peppers (bell peppers), de-seeded and finely chopped

2 tablespoons light crème fraîche

600mls (1 pint) hot vegetable stock (broth)

Sea salt

Freshly ground black pepper

SERVES 2

76 calories per serving

Method

Place the red peppers (bell peppers) into a saucepan and pour in the hot stock (broth). Bring the ingredients to the boil, reduce the heat and simmer for a few minutes until the pepper has softened. Using a hand blender or food processor blitz the soup until smooth. Stir in the crème fraîche and season with salt and pepper. Serve and enjoy.

Tomato & Basil Soup

Ingredients

2 x 400g (14oz) tins of chopped tomatoes

1 onion, peeled and chopped

1 small handful of fresh basil, chopped

600mls (1 pint) vegetable stock (broth)

1 tablespoon olive oil

Sea salt

Freshly ground black pepper

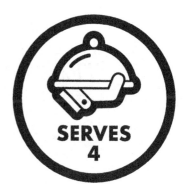

SERVES 4

90
calories
per serving

Method

Heat the oil in a saucepan, add the onion and cook for 5 minutes until the onion has softened, Add the tomatoes and stock (broth) and bring it to the boil. Reduce the heat and simmer for 5 minutes. Using a food processor and or hand blender blitz until smooth. Add in the basil. Season with salt and pepper. Serve and enjoy.

Creamy Tomato & Pesto Soup

Ingredients

6 large tomatoes

2 stalks of celery, chopped

2 teaspoons pesto

1 tablespoon crème fraîche

600mls (1 pint) hot stock (broth)

Freshly ground black pepper

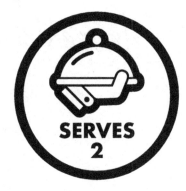

SERVES 2

84 calories per serving

Method

Place the tomatoes, celery and pesto into a saucepan and add the stock (broth). Cook for 8-10 minutes. Using a hand blender or food processor, blitz the soup until it's smooth. Add the crème fraîche and stir well. Season with salt and pepper then serve.

Garlic Mushroom Wraps

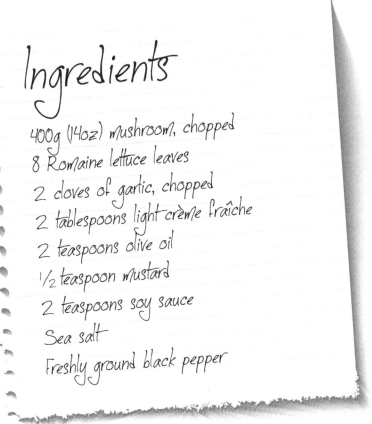

Ingredients

400g (14oz) mushroom, chopped

8 Romaine lettuce leaves

2 cloves of garlic, chopped

2 tablespoons light crème fraîche

2 teaspoons olive oil

½ teaspoon mustard

2 teaspoons soy sauce

Sea salt

Freshly ground black pepper

SERVES 2

99
calories
per serving

Method

Heat the oil in a frying pan, add the mushrooms, garlic, mustard and soy sauce and cook for around 5 minutes or until the mushrooms have softened. Stir in the crème fraîche and warm it thoroughly. Season with salt and pepper. Spoon some of the mixture into each of the lettuce leaves and eat straight away.

Carrot & Apple Smoothie

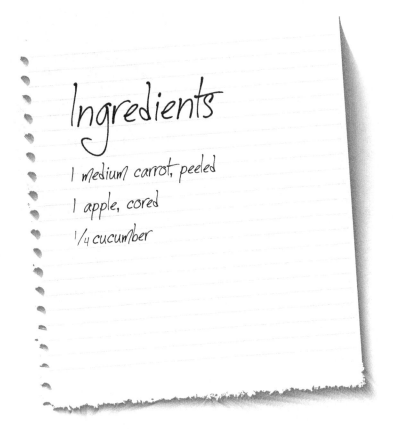

Ingredients

1 medium carrot, peeled

1 apple, cored

¼ cucumber

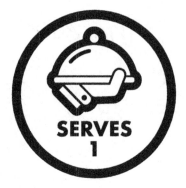

**SERVES
1**

78
calories
per serving

Method

Place all the ingredients into a blender and add around a cup of water. Blitz until smooth.
You can add a little extra water if it's too thick.

Cauliflower 'Rice'

Ingredients

1 head of cauliflower, approx. 700g (1½ lb)

1 tablespoon olive oil

Sea salt

Freshly ground black pepper

SERVES 4

81 calories per serving

Method

Place the cauliflower into a food processor and chop until fine, similar to rice. Heat the olive oil in a frying pan, stir in the cauliflower and cook for 5-6 minutes or until softened. Season with salt and pepper. Serve with meat or vegetable dishes as a tasty alternative to rice.

Recipes Under 200 Calories

Breakfast Muffins

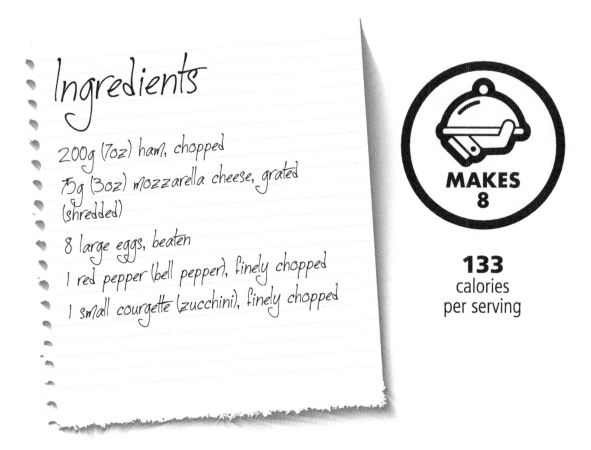

Ingredients

- 200g (7oz) ham, chopped
- 75g (3oz) mozzarella cheese, grated (shredded)
- 8 large eggs, beaten
- 1 red pepper (bell pepper), finely chopped
- 1 small courgette (zucchini), finely chopped

MAKES 8

133 calories per serving

Method

Combine the beaten eggs with the ham, mozzarella, red pepper (bell pepper) and courgette (zucchini). Place paper cases inside an 8–hole muffin tin. Spoon the egg mixture into the cases. Transfer them to the oven and bake at 180C/360F for 20 minutes or until the eggs are completely set. These can be eaten hot or cold.

Cheese & Ham Breakfast Peppers

Ingredients

25g (1oz) mozzarella cheese, grated (shredded)

2 red peppers (bell peppers), cut in half and de-seeded

2 slices ham, cut in half

2 eggs, beaten

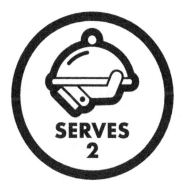

SERVES 2

160 calories per serving

Method

Place a slice of ham into each pepper half. Pour some of the beaten egg into each of the pepper halves. Place the mozzarella on top. Transfer the peppers to a baking sheet and cook in the oven at 190C/375F for 25 minutes or until the eggs have set.

Pink Grapefruit & Carrot Smoothie

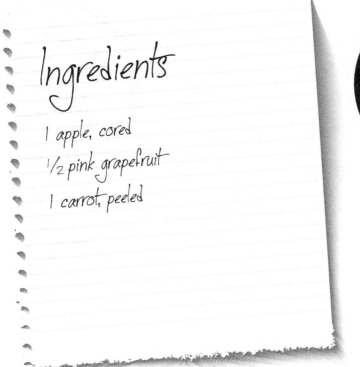

Ingredients

1 apple, cored

1/2 pink grapefruit

1 carrot, peeled

SERVES 1

137 calories per serving

Method

Place all the ingredients into a blender with enough water to cover them and blitz until smooth.

Carrot, Coriander & Butterbean Soup

Ingredients

400g (14oz) butter beans
4 carrots, chopped
1 onion, chopped
1 courgette (zucchini), chopped
1 clove of garlic, chopped
900mls (1½ pints) vegetable stock (broth)
1 handful of fresh coriander (cilantro), chopped
Sea salt
Freshly ground black pepper

SERVES 4

159
calories
per serving

Method

Heat the vegetable stock (broth) in a large saucepan. Add in all of the vegetables except the coriander and butterbeans. Bring them to the boil, reduce the heat and simmer for 20 minutes. Add the butterbeans and stir until warmed through. Add in half of the chopped coriander (cilantro). Using a hand blender or food processor, process the soup until smooth. Sprinkle with the remaining coriander and serve.

Cream Of Mushroom Soup

Ingredients

450g (1lb) mushrooms, chopped

1 large leek, finely chopped

1 tablespoon cornflour (corn starch)

750mls (1¼ pints) vegetable stock (broth)

4 tablespoons crème fraîche

1 tablespoon olive oil

Sea salt

Freshly ground black pepper

SERVES 4

120
calories
per serving

Method

Heat the olive oil in a saucepan. Add the leek and mushrooms and cook for 8 minutes or until the vegetables are soft. Sprinkle in the cornflour (corn starch) and stir. Pour in the stock (broth), bring it to the boil, cover and simmer for 20 minutes. Stir in the crème fraîche. Using a hand blender or food processor, blend the soup until smooth. Return to the heat if necessary. Season with salt and pepper just before serving.

Asparagus Soup

Ingredients

900g (2lbs) asparagus spears, tough end of stalk removed

2 tablespoons light crème fraîche

1 onion, chopped

1 tablespoon olive oil

900mls (1½ pints) vegetable stock (broth)

Sea salt

Freshly ground black pepper

SERVES 4

139 calories per serving

Method

Heat the oil in a large saucepan, add the onion and cook for 5 minutes. Break off the tough root end of the asparagus and discard it. Roughly chop the asparagus spears. Place them in the saucepan and add the stock (broth). Bring it to the boil, reduce the heat and simmer for 20 minutes Using a food processor or hand blender process the soup until smooth and creamy. Stir in the crème fraîche. Season and serve.

Chicken & Mushroom Soup

Ingredients

100g (3½ oz) cooked chicken, chopped

4 large mushrooms, finely sliced

6 spring onions (scallions), finely chopped

2 sticks of celery, finely chopped

2 teaspoons olive oil

600mls (1 pint) chicken stock (broth)

Sea salt

Freshly ground black pepper

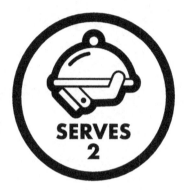

SERVES 2

144 calories per serving

Method

Heat the oil in a saucepan, add the mushrooms, spring onions (scallions) and celery and cook for 3-4 minutes. Pour in the stock (broth) and chopped chicken. Bring it to the boil, reduce the heat and cook for 10 minutes. Season with salt and pepper.

Mozzarella Slices

Ingredients

300g (11oz) mozzarella cheese, grated (shredded)

4 eggs, beaten

3 cloves of garlic, crushed

2 teaspoons dried oregano

1 cauliflower (approx. 700g), grated (shredded)

Sea salt

Freshly ground black pepper

SERVES 8

157 calories per serving

Method

Place the cauliflower into a steamer and cook for 5 minutes. Place the cauliflower in a bowl and combine it with the mozzarella, eggs, oregano and garlic. Season with salt and pepper. Grease 2 baking sheets. Divide the mixture in half and place it on the baking sheet and press it into a flat rectangular shape. Preheat the oven to 220C/440F. Transfer the baking sheets to the oven and cook for for 20-25 minutes and golden. Slice and serve.

Tomato & Olive Salad

Ingredients

150g (5oz) cherry tomatoes, halved

75g (3oz) black olives, chopped

50g (2oz) capers

1 romaine lettuce, chopped

1 cucumber chopped

1 red pepper (bell pepper), sliced

1 onion, sliced

2 tablespoons red wine vinegar

1 tablespoon freshly squeezed lemon juice

1/2 teaspoon dried oregano

1/4 teaspoon dried basil

3 tablespoons olive oil

Sea salt

Freshly ground black pepper

SERVES 4

176 calories per serving

Method

Pour the vinegar into a large bowl and add in the olive oil, lemon juice, basil and oregano and mix well. Season with salt and pepper. Add the tomatoes, olives, capers, lettuce, cucumber, red pepper (bell pepper) and onion. Toss the salad ingredients in the dressing.

Baked Cod

Ingredients

2 skinless cod fillets

4 stalks of celery, chopped

2 teaspoon fresh parsley, chopped

2 teaspoon fresh coriander (cilantro), chopped

2 tablespoon fresh lemon juice

Sea salt

Freshly ground black pepper

**SERVES
2**

125
calories
per serving

Method

Place the celery into an ovenproof dish and add the lemon juice, parsley and coriander (cilantro). Lay the fish on top of the vegetables and season with salt and pepper then cover the dish. Transfer the dish to the oven and cook at 200C/400F for 20 minutes or until the fish is completely cooked. Serve and eat straight away.

Prawn Skewers

Ingredients

10 large king prawns (shrimp), peeled

4 cherry tomatoes

4 pitted black olives

1 tablespoon fresh coriander (cilantro) leaves, chopped

1 teaspoon olive oil

Rind and juice of a lemon

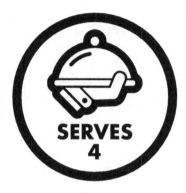

SERVES 4

124
calories
per serving

Method

Place the oil, coriander (cilantro), olives and lemon juice in a bowl and stir well. Add the prawns to the bowl and coat them in the mixture. Thread the prawns, tomatoes and olives alternately onto 2 skewers. Place the skewers under a hot grill (broiler) and cook until the prawns are completely pink throughout. Serve on their own or with a leafy salad.

Mediterranean Fried 'Rice'

Ingredients

200g (7oz) mushrooms, finely chopped

6 spring onions (scallions), finely chopped

1 head of cauliflower, approx. 700g (1½ lb) broken into florets

1 red pepper (bell pepper), peeled and finely chopped

1 onion, finely chopped

1 large egg, beaten

2 tablespoons olive oil

2 tablespoons soy sauce

Sea salt

Freshly ground black pepper

SERVES 4

149 calories per serving

Method

Place the cauliflower pieces into a food processor and chop until it becomes grain-like. In a bowl mix together the egg with a tablespoon of soy sauce. Heat a tablespoon of oil in a large frying pan or wok. Add the egg mixture and scramble it for a few minutes then remove it and set aside. Heat the remaining olive oil and add in the red onion and cook for 5 minutes. Add in all the remaining vegetables and cook them for around 5 minutes until they soften. Stir in the remaining soy sauce. Add the cooked egg mixture and stir well. Season with salt and pepper. Serve instead of traditional fried rice.

Parmesan Chicken & Asparagus

Ingredients

350g (12oz) asparagus spears, trimmed

25g (1oz) Parmesan cheese, grated

4 chicken breasts

4 cloves of garlic, chopped

2 red peppers (bell peppers), deseeded and chopped

2 tomatoes, chopped

2 tablespoons fresh basil, chopped

2 tablespoons fresh parsley, chopped

2 tablespoons fresh tarragon, chopped

1 tablespoon capers, drained

Zest of 1 lemon

2 tablespoons olive oil

SERVES 4

176 calories per serving

Method

Preheat the oven to 200C/400F. Place the herbs, garlic, capers and olive oil into a food processor and blitz to combine them. Combine the mixture with the lemon zest and parmesan. Spread the topping onto the chicken breasts. Add the chicken to a roasting tin. Place it in the oven and cook for 10 minutes. Add in the asparagus, red peppers (bell peppers) and tomatoes. Return it to the oven and cook for 10-15 minutes or until the vegetables have softened and the chicken is completely cooked.

Spinach & Herb Stuffed Chicken

Ingredients

- 4 chicken breasts
- 4 tablespoons cream cheese
- 25g (1oz) spinach leaves
- 1 tablespoon fresh parsley
- 1 tablespoon fresh chives

SERVES 4

192 calories per serving

Method

In a bowl, combine the cream cheese, spinach and herbs until it's well mixed. Carefully make an incision on the underside of the chicken breast, wide enough to contain some cheese mixture. Spoon some of the mixture into the incision and press the chicken back together. Repeat for the remaining mixture. Place the stuffed chicken in an ovenproof dish. Transfer to the oven and bake at 180C/360F for around 30 minutes or until the chicken is completely cooked. Serve with a large green leafy salad. Enjoy.

Sea Bass & Ratatouille

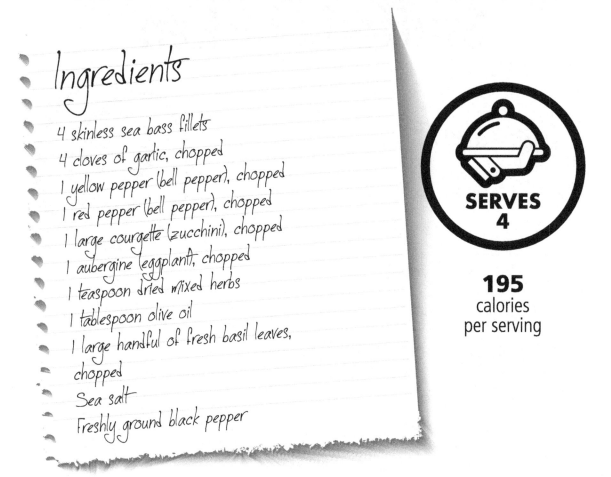

Ingredients

4 skinless sea bass fillets
4 cloves of garlic, chopped
1 yellow pepper (bell pepper), chopped
1 red pepper (bell pepper), chopped
1 large courgette (zucchini), chopped
1 aubergine (eggplant), chopped
1 teaspoon dried mixed herbs
1 tablespoon olive oil
1 large handful of fresh basil leaves, chopped
Sea salt
Freshly ground black pepper

SERVES 4

195 calories per serving

Method

Place the courgette (zucchini) aubergine (eggplant), peppers, garlic, mixed herbs and oil, into an ovenproof roasting dish and toss them well. Season with salt and pepper. Transfer it to the oven and cook at 200C/400F for 25 minutes. Add in half of the fresh basil and stir the vegetables. Place the fish on top of the vegetables. Return it to the oven and cook for 10-12 minutes or until the fish is completely cooked and flakes off. Sprinkle the remaining basil on top and serve.

Baked Eggs & Peppers

Ingredients

4 eggs

1 red pepper (bell pepper), chopped

1 green pepper (bell pepper), chopped

1 large aubergine (eggplant, chopped

1 bulb of fennel, chopped

1 onion, chopped

3 cloves of garlic, chopped

1 handful of fresh basil

2 tablespoons olive oil

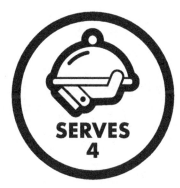

**SERVES
4**

174
calories
per serving

Method

Place all the vegetables, garlic and basil in a large ovenproof dish. Pour in the olive oil and toss the vegetables. Transfer it to the oven and cook at 200C/400F for 20 minutes. Make 4 round indentations in the vegetables and crack an egg into each space. Place the dish back into the oven and cook for 10 minutes. Serve and eat immediately.

Roast Courgettes & Olives

Ingredients

10 pitted black olives, chopped

4 medium courgettes (zucchinis), thickly sliced lengthways

2 tablespoons tomato purée (paste)

1 clove of garlic, crushed

1 teaspoon mixed herbs

2 tablespoons olive oil

Sea salt

Freshly ground black pepper

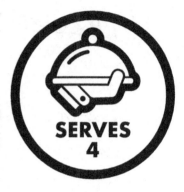

SERVES 4

107 calories per serving

Method

In a bowl, combine the olive oil, garlic, tomato purée (paste) and mixed herbs. Place the courgette (zucchini) slices in an ovenproof dish and spread the oil mixture over the slices. Sprinkle with olives and season with salt and pepper. Transfer them to an oven, preheated to 200C/400F and cook for 15 minutes.

Recipes Under 300 Calories

Cheese & Tomato Mini Cauliflower Pizzas

Ingredients

- 350g (12 oz) mozzarella cheese, grated (shredded)
- 200g (7oz) passata/ tomato sauce
- 2 eggs
- 1 head of cauliflower approx. 700g (1½ lb), grated (shredded)
- 1 teaspoon dried oregano
- 1 teaspoon dried basil
- 1 teaspoon garlic powder
- 1 tomato, sliced
- Handful of fresh basil leaves, chopped

SERVES 6

219
calories
per serving

Method

Steam the grated (shredded) cauliflower for 5 minutes then allow it to cool. Place the cooked cauliflower in a bowl and add the eggs, half the cheese, all of the dried herbs and garlic and mix everything together really well. Grease two baking sheets. Divide the mixture into 12 and roll it into balls. Place them on a baking sheet and press them down until are flat and round mini pizza bases. Transfer them to the oven and bake at 220C/440F for 12 minutes until lightly golden. Top each pizza base with a little passata, the remaining mozzarella and tomato and fresh basil. Place the pizzas under a grill (broiler) and cook for 4-5 minutes or until the cheese has melted. Enjoy.

Tomato & Olive Stuffed Chicken

Ingredients

450g (1lb) chicken breasts

75g (3oz) black olives, finely chopped

25g (1oz) butter, softened

6 sundried tomatoes, finely chopped

3 cloves of garlic, crushed

1 tablespoon capers

1 teaspoon dried oregano

1 teaspoon dried basil

Sea salt

Freshly ground black pepper

SERVES 4

287
calories
per serving

Method

Place the olives, tomatoes, garlic, dried herbs and capers into a bowl and stir. Add in the softened butter and capers and mix well. Make an incision in each chicken breast to make a pocket for the butter mixture. Spoon the mixture inside each of the chicken breasts. Season with salt and pepper and wrap each one in tin foil. Transfer them to the oven and cook at 190C/375F for 25 minutes.

Prawn Oven Traybake

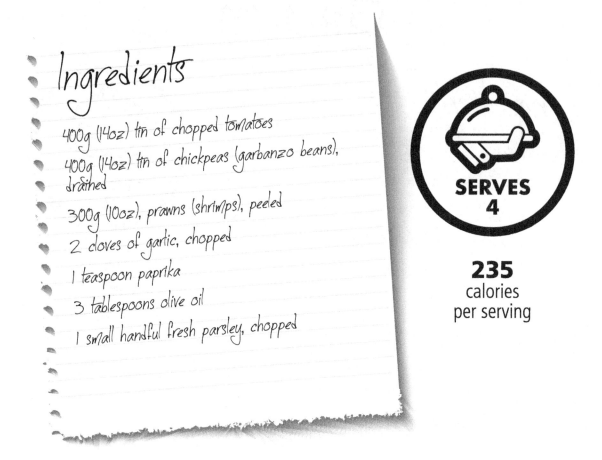

Ingredients

400g (14oz) tin of chopped tomatoes

400g (14oz) tin of chickpeas (garbanzo beans), drained

300g (10oz), prawns (shrimps), peeled

2 cloves of garlic, chopped

1 teaspoon paprika

3 tablespoons olive oil

1 small handful fresh parsley, chopped

SERVES 4

235 calories per serving

Method

Heat the oven to 190C/380F. Scatter the chickpeas (garbanzo beans), tomatoes, garlic and paprika into an oven proof dish. Add in the olive oil and mix well. Transfer it to the oven and cook for 10 minutes. Scatter the prawns into the dish, return it to the oven and cook for around 10 minutes or until the prawns are pink and completely cooked through. Sprinkle with parsley.

Lemon & Coriander (Cilantro) Chicken

Ingredients

450g (1lb) chicken breasts
1 onion, finely chopped
3 cloves of garlic, crushed
2 lemons, sliced and pips removed
1 teaspoon ground coriander (cilantro)
1 teaspoon ground ginger
1 teaspoon ground cumin
1 teaspoon ground turmeric
1 tablespoon olive oil
600mls (1 pint) chicken stock (broth)
125g (4oz) pitted green olives
Handful of fresh coriander (cilantro) finely chopped

SERVES 4

278 calories per serving

Method

Heat the oil in a saucepan, add the onion and cook for 5 minutes until softened. Add the garlic, cumin, turmeric, ginger and ground coriander (cilantro) and cook for 1 minute. Add the chicken and brown it. Add the slices of lemon and chicken stock (broth). Bring it to the boil, reduce the heat and simmer for 30 minutes. Stir in the fresh coriander (cilantro) and olives. Warm the olives through and then serve.

Chilli Chicken Skewers & Roast Cauliflower

Ingredients

450g (1lb) chicken breast, diced

12 cherry tomatoes

1 large cauliflower

1 onion, peeled and chopped

1 teaspoon smoked paprika

1/2 teaspoon mild chilli powder

2 tablespoons olive oil

Sea salt

Freshly ground black pepper

SERVES 4

292
calories
per serving

Method

Preheat the oven to 180C/360F. Place the chicken into a large bowl and add the chilli and smoked paprika and a tablespoon of olive oil. Coat the chicken completely in the mixture. Add a tablespoon of olive oil to a large roasting tin. Cut the cauliflower into slices. Scatter them in the roasting tin, together with the onion and coat them in olive oil. Thread the chicken chunks onto skewers, alternating them with the tomatoes. Lay the chicken skewers in top of the cauliflower and season with salt and pepper. Transfer the roasting tin to the oven and cook for 25-30 minutes or until the chicken is completely cooked and the cauliflower is tender. Serve and eat straight away.

Mediterranean Vegetable Bake

Ingredients

400g (14oz) cannellini beans

150g (5oz) cherry tomatoes, halved

150g (5oz) button mushrooms

3 cloves of garlic, peeled and chopped

3 celery stalks, chopped

3 medium carrots, peeled and roughly chopped

1 large onion, peeled and chopped

1 butternut squash, peeled and cut into chunks

1 courgette (zucchini), chopped

1 teaspoon dried thyme

1 teaspoon dried oregano

1 large handful of fresh basil

A small handful of fresh parsley, chopped

2 tablespoons olive oil

Sea salt

Freshly ground black pepper

SERVES 4

295 calories per serving

Method

Place the beans and vegetables into a roasting tin. Sprinkle in the dried herbs, garlic and olive oil and toss all of the ingredients together. Season with salt and pepper. Transfer them to an oven, preheated to 180C/360F and cook for 30-40 minutes or until all of the vegetables are softened. Scatter in the fresh parsley just before serving.

Garlic Chicken & Pepper Skewers

SERVES 4

275 calories per serving

Ingredients

450g (1lb) chicken breasts, cut into chunks

4 cloves of garlic, finely chopped

1 teaspoon dried oregano

1 red pepper (bell pepper) cut into 2cm (1 inch) chunks

1 yellow pepper (bell pepper) cut into 2cm (1 inch chunks)

1 onion, peeled and cut into 2cm (1 inch) chunks

2 tablespoon olive oil

2 tablespoons soy sauce

Juice of 1/2 lime

1 small handful of fresh parsley, chopped

Method

Place the olive oil, soy sauce, lime, oregano and garlic into a large bowl and mix well. Add the in the chicken, bell peppers and onion to the bowl. Toss the ingredients in the oil mixture. Cover and refrigerate for at least 1 hour. Thread the chicken, onion and peppers onto skewers. If using wooden skewers, soak them for 30 minutes beforehand. Place the skewers under a hot grill (broiler). Cook for 5-7 minutes on each side until the chicken is completely cooked through. Sprinkle with parsley and serve.

Easy Banana Pancakes

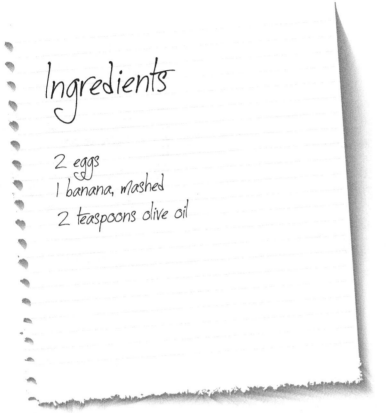

Ingredients

2 eggs
1 banana, mashed
2 teaspoons olive oil

**SERVES
1**

297
calories
per serving

Method

Whisk the eggs in a bowl and stir in the mashed banana. Combine them until the mixture is smooth. Heat the olive oil in a frying pan, add the pancake mixture and cook for around 2 minutes on each side or until the batter has set and the pancakes are golden. Serve and eat immediately. You can even add a little butter and a sprinkling of cinnamon on top.

Cheese & Mushroom Chops

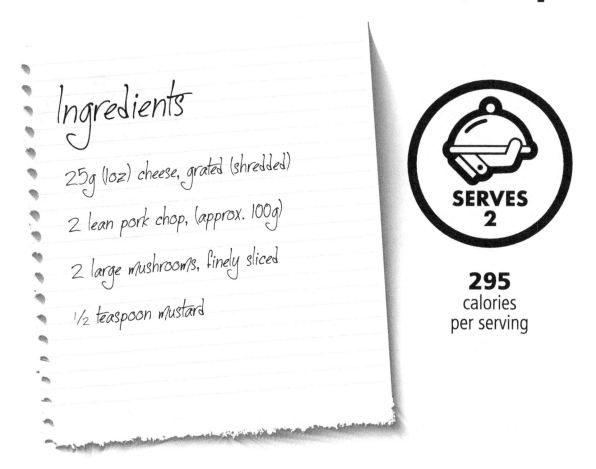

Ingredients

25g (1oz) cheese, grated (shredded)

2 lean pork chop, (approx. 100g)

2 large mushrooms, finely sliced

½ teaspoon mustard

SERVES 2

295 calories per serving

Method

Place the pork chop under a preheated grill (broiler) and cook for 6 minutes. Turn the chop over and cook on the other side for 6 minutes. Spread a little mustard over the chop. Lay the mushroom slices over the chop and scatter the grated (shredded) cheese on top. Return the chops to the grill and cook until the cheese is bubbling.

Bean & Quinoa Casserole

Ingredients

450g (1lb) black-eyed beans, drained

200g (7oz) frozen peas

100g (3½ oz) fresh spinach leaves

100g (3½ oz) quinoa

2 x 400g (14oz) tins of chopped tomatoes

2 cloves garlic, chopped

1 red onion, chopped

1 teaspoon cumin

1 teaspoon dried oregano

½ teaspoon chilli powder

125mls (4fl oz) water

1 tablespoon olive oil

SERVES 4

292 calories per serving

Method

Heat the oil in a saucepan, add the onion and garlic and cook for 5 minutes. Transfer to an ovenproof dish. Add in the quinoa, tomatoes, cumin, oregano and chilli powder. Place the dish in the oven and cook at 180C/360F for 20 minutes. Stir in the beans, peas and water. Cover with foil and cook for 20 minutes. Remove it from the oven, stir in the spinach and allow it to wilt for a couple of minutes before serving.

Courgette Fritters

Ingredients

- 450g (1lb) courgettes (zucchinis), grated (shredded)
- 100g (3½ oz) Parmesan cheese
- 3 cloves of garlic, chopped
- 3 spring onions (scallions)
- 2 eggs
- 1 teaspoon dried mixed herbs
- 1 tablespoon olive oil
- Sprinkling of salt

SERVES 4

204 calories per serving

Method

Place the grated (shredded) courgette (zucchini) into a colander and sprinkle with a little salt. Allow it to sit for 30 minutes then squeeze out any excess moisture. Place the eggs, Parmesan, spring onions (scallions), garlic and dried herbs into a bowl and mix well with the courgettes. Scoop out a spoonful of the mixture and shape it into patties. Repeat for the remaining mixture. Heat the oil in a frying pan, add the patties and cook for 2 minutes, turn them over and cook for another 2 minutes. Serve warm.

Mozzarella & Tomato Mug Omelette

Ingredients

25g (1oz) mozzarella cheese

2 cherry tomatoes, chopped

2 eggs

2 teaspoons chopped red pepper (bell pepper)

1/2 teaspoon dried oregano

1/4 teaspoon softened butter

SERVES 1

221
calories
per serving

Method

Crack the eggs into a large mug and beat them. Add in the remaining ingredients. Place the mug in a microwave and cook on full power for 30 seconds. Stir and return it to the microwave for another 30 seconds, stir and cook for another 30-60 seconds or until the egg is set. Alternatively, try plain eggs as a quick and easy alternative to scrambling.

Herby Ham
& Cheese Omelette

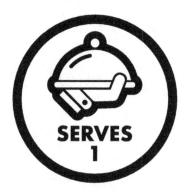

**SERVES
1**

254
calories
per serving

Ingredients

25g (1oz) goats cheese, crumbled

1 slice of ham (chopped)

2 eggs

½ teaspoon softened butter

1 teaspoon fresh basil, chopped

Method

Whisk the eggs in a large mug. Add in the cheese, ham, basil and butter. Place the mug in a microwave and cook on full power for 30 seconds. Stir and return it to the microwave for another 30 seconds, stir and cook for another 30-60 seconds or until the egg is completely set. Enjoy straight from the mug.

Tomato & Basil Eggs

Ingredients

400g (14oz) tinned chopped tomatoes

4 large eggs, beaten

1 small handful of fresh basil leaves, chopped

1 tablespoon olive oil

Sea salt

Freshly ground black pepper

SERVES 2

252
calories
per serving

Method

Heat the olive oil in a pan and add in the chopped tomatoes. Cook for around
10 minutes to reduce the tomato mixture down until the excess juice has evaporated.
Slowly pour in the beaten egg, stirring constantly until the egg is completely cooked.
Season and sprinkle with basil before serving.

Aubergine Fries

Ingredients

125g (4oz) ground almonds (almond meal /almond flour)

1 large egg

1 large aubergine (eggplant, cut lengthwise into batons

½ teaspoon salt

½ teaspoon ground cumin

½ teaspoon paprika

1 tablespoon olive oil

Sea salt

Freshly ground black pepper

SERVES 4

255 calories per serving

Method

Place the ground almonds on a large plate and season with salt and pepper. In a bowl, beat the egg and stir in the cumin and paprika and oil. Dip the aubergine batons in egg mixture then roll them in the almond mixture. Place the aubergine on a baking sheet. Transfer it to the oven and cook at 220C/425F for 15 minutes.

Egg & Lentil Salad

Ingredients

200g (7oz) Puy lentils

4 eggs

4 tomatoes, deseeded and chopped

4 spring onions (scallions), finely chopped

2 tablespoons olive oil

2 tablespoons parsley

2 large handfuls of washed spinach leaves

1 clove of garlic

Juice and rind of 1 lemon

Sea salt

Freshly ground black pepper

SERVES 4

231 calories per serving

Method

Place the lentils in a saucepan, cover them with water and bring them to the boil. Reduce the heat and cook for 20-25 minutes. Drain them once they are soft. Heat the olive oil in a saucepan, add the garlic and spring onions (scallions) and cook for 2 minutes. Stir in the tomatoes, lemon juice and rind. Cook for 2 minutes. Stir in the lentils and keep warm. In a pan of gently simmering water, poach the eggs until they are set but soft in the middle which should be 3-4 minutes. Scatter the spinach leaves onto plates, serve the lentils and top off with a poached egg. Season with salt and pepper. Sprinkle with parsley and serve.

Mixed Bean Salad

Ingredients

- 100g (3½ oz) tinned mixed beans, drained
- 1 hard-boiled egg, quartered
- 1 medium tomato, chopped
- 1 spring onion (scallion), finely chopped
- 2 teaspoon olive oil
- 1 small handful of fresh basil, chopped
- 1 large handful of fresh spinach
- 1 clove of garlic, finely chopped
- Zest and juice of 1 lime
- Sea salt
- Freshly ground black pepper

SERVES 1

266 calories per serving

Method

Heat the oil in a frying pan, add the garlic and spring onions (scallions) and cook for 2 minutes. Stir in the mixed beans, tomato, lime zest and juice. Cook for 3 minutes until the tomatoes are warmed. Stir in the fresh basil and season with salt and pepper. Scatter the spinach leaves onto a plate and serve the lentil mixture on top. Lay the egg on top. Serve and eat straight away.

Mozzarella Roast Vegetables

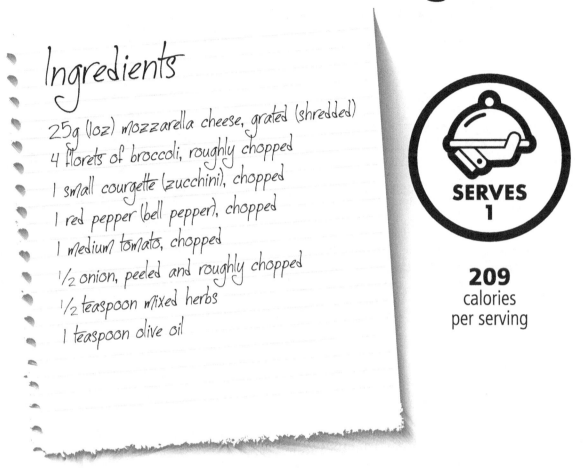

Ingredients

25g (1oz) mozzarella cheese, grated (shredded)
4 florets of broccoli, roughly chopped
1 small courgette (zucchini), chopped
1 red pepper (bell pepper), chopped
1 medium tomato, chopped
1/2 onion, peeled and roughly chopped
1/2 teaspoon mixed herbs
1 teaspoon olive oil

**SERVES
1**

209
calories
per serving

Method

Place all of the ingredients, apart from the mozzarella, into a large ovenproof dish and mix them well. Place the vegetables in the oven and cook them at 200C/400F for 20 minutes. Remove the dish from the oven and sprinkle over the mozzarella cheese. Return it to the oven and continue cooking for 5-10 minutes when the cheese is completely melted. Use as a side dish to go along with chicken, meat and fish meals instead of potatoes or pasta.

Halloumi & Asparagus Salad

SERVES 4

257
calories
per serving

Ingredients

450g (1lb) asparagus

250g (9oz) halloumi cheese, cut into slices

2 large handfuls of spinach leaves

1 tablespoon olive oil

Sea salt

Freshly ground black pepper

Method

Heat the olive oil in a frying pan and cook the asparagus for 4 minutes or until tender. Remove, set aside and keep warm. Place the halloumi in the frying pan and cook for 2 minutes on each side until golden. Serve the spinach leaves onto plates and add the asparagus and halloumi slices. Season with salt and pepper.

Courgette 'Spaghetti' Pesto & Avocado Dressing

Ingredients

1 medium courgette (zucchini)

1/2 ripe avocado, peeled and stone removed

1 teaspoon pesto sauce

1 teaspoon olive oilive oil

1 teaspoon lemon juice

SERVES 1

231
calories
per serving

Method

Use a spiraliser or if you don't have one, use a vegetable peeler and cut the courgette (zucchini) into thin strips. Heat a teaspoon of oil in a frying pan, add the courgette (zucchini) and cook for 4-5 minutes or until it has softened. In the meantime, place the avocado, pesto and lemon juice and a teaspoon of olive oil into a blender and process until smooth. Add the avocado mixture to the courgette (zucchini) and stir it well. Serve and eat straight away.

Mediterranean Cod

Ingredients

400g (14oz) tin of chopped tomatoes

75g (3oz) pitted black olives, sliced

4 cod fillets

1 onion, chopped

2 cloves of garlic, crushed

2 tablespoons olive oil

100mls (3½ fl oz) vegetable or chicken stock (broth)

A small handful of fresh parsley

SERVES 4

223
calories
per serving

Method

Heat the oil in a frying pan, add the onions and garlic and cook for 5 minutes. Add in chopped tomatoes, parsley, olives and stock. Bring it to the boil and simmer for 5 minutes. Add the cod fillets to the tomato sauce and simmer for 5-6 minutes or until the fish flakes and is completely cooked.

Chicken & Quinoa Salad

Ingredients

450g (1lb) chicken breasts, cooked and sliced

125g (4oz) quinoa, cooked

50g (2oz) fresh spinach leaves, chopped

8 spring onions (scallions), chopped

1 handful fresh coriander (cilantro), chopped

1 handful fresh parsley, chopped

2 tomatoes, diced

1 cucumber, peeled and diced

1 teaspoon ground turmeric

2 tablespoons olive oil

Juice of 1 lime

Sea salt

Freshly ground black pepper

SERVES 4

296 calories per serving

Method

Combine all of the ingredients in a large bowl and mix well. Season with salt and pepper. Cover and place in the fridge for 20 minutes to chill before serving.

Tuna Casserole

Ingredients

- 4 tuna steaks
- 2 red onions, chopped
- 2 stalks of celery
- 2 x 400g (2 x 14oz) tins of chopped tomatoes
- 2 cloves of garlic
- 1 tablespoon olive oil
- 1 lemon, thinly sliced
- 1 tablespoon tomato purée (paste)
- 1 small handful of fresh oregano, chopped
- Sea salt
- Freshly ground black pepper

SERVES 4

229
calories
per serving

Method

Heat the oil in a saucepan and add the celery, garlic and onions and fry for 5 minutes until the vegetables have softened. Add in the tinned tomatoes, oregano, tomato purée (paste) and lemon slices. Bring to the boil and simmer for 5 minutes, stirring occasionally. Season with salt and pepper. Place the fish in the tomato mixture. Simmer gently for 12-14 minutes until the fish is cooked. Serve the fish onto plates and pour the sauce on top. Garnish with some fresh oregano.

Recipes Under 400 Calories

Steak & Cheese Lettuce Wraps

Ingredients

450g (1lb) lean minced steak (ground steak)

75g (3oz) cheese, grated (shredded)

4 tomatoes, sliced

1 tablespoon tomato purée (paste)

1 romaine lettuce, leaves washed and separated

1 teaspoon dried cumin

1 teaspoon paprika

1/2 teaspoon dried oregano

1 tablespoons olive oil

SERVES 4

326 calories per serving

Method

Heat the olive oil in a frying pan, add the steak, cumin, paprika and oregano and cook for 10 minutes. Add in the tomato purée (paste) and cook for another 5 minutes until the meat is completely cooked. Lay out the lettuce leaves and spoon some meat into each one. Add the tomato slices and sprinkle with cheese. Serve and eat immediately.

Olive, Tomato & Herb Frittata

Ingredients

- 50g (2oz) mozzarella cheese, grated (shredded)
- 75g (3oz) pitted black olives, halved
- 8 cherry tomatoes, halved
- 4 large eggs
- 1 small handful of fresh parsley, chopped
- 1 small handful of fresh basil leaves, chopped
- 1 tablespoon olive oil

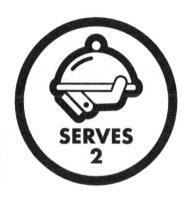

SERVES 2

343 calories per serving

Method

Break the eggs into a bowl and whisk them then add in the parsley, basil, olives and tomatoes. Add in the cheese and stir it. Heat the oil in a small frying pan and pour in the egg mixture. Cook until the egg mixture completely sets. Place the frittata under a hot grill for 3 minutes to finish it off. Carefully remove it from the pan. Cut into slices and serve.

Chilli Mushroom & Bean Omelette

Ingredients

50g (2oz) tinned cannellini beans, drained

50g (2oz) mushrooms, chopped

2 eggs

1 red pepper (bell pepper)

1 tablespoon olive oil

Dash of Tabasco sauce or a sprinkle of chilli powder

SERVES 1

341 calories per serving

Method

Heat the olive oil in a pan. Add the mushrooms, pepper (bell pepper) and beans. Cook for 3-4 minutes until the vegetables have softened. Remove them and set aside. Whisk the eggs in a bowl and pour them into the pan. Once the eggs begin to set, return the mushrooms, peppers and beans and spread them onto the eggs. Sprinkle with chilli or Tabasco sauce. Serve and eat straight away.

Fresh Basil, Mozzarella & Tomato Chicken

Ingredients

4 chicken breasts

2 x 400g (14oz) tinned chopped tomatoes

125g (4oz) mozzarella cheese, sliced

600mls (1 pint) vegetable stock (broth)

1 large handful of fresh basil leaves, torn

2 cloves of garlic, chopped

1 onion chopped

1 tablespoon olive oil

SERVES 4

324
calories
per serving

Method

Heat the olive oil in a frying pan, add the onion and garlic and cook for 5 minutes or until softened. Add the chopped tomatoes and stock (broth). Add in the basil leaves, bring it to the boil, reduce the heat and simmer for 5 minutes. Place the chicken in an ovenproof dish. Cover the chicken with the sauce and add slices of mozzarella to the dish on top of the chicken. Transfer it to the oven and cook at 190C/375F for around 20 minutes or until the chicken is completely cooked. Serve with a leafy green salad.

Cheese & Courgette Omelette

Ingredients

- 25g (1oz) feta cheese, crumbled
- 2 eggs
- 1 small courgette (zucchini), grated (shredded)
- 1 teaspoon fresh parsley, chopped
- 1 tablespoon olive oil

SERVES 1

337 calories per serving

Method

Place the eggs in a bowl and whisk them. Stir in the cheese and courgette (zucchini). Heat the olive oil in a frying pan. Pour in the egg mixture and cook until it is set. Sprinkle with parsley and serve.

Creamy Lime & Mint Smoothie

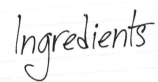

Ingredients

250mls (8fl oz) coconut water

8 fresh mint leaves

1 medium avocado, stone and skin removed

Juice of 1/2 lime

**SERVES
1**

323
calories
per serving

Method

Place the ingredients into a blender and blitz until smooth.

Piri Piri Prawn Salad

Ingredients

- 16 king prawns (shrimps), peeled
- 2 handfuls of mixed lettuce leaves
- 2 tomatoes, chopped
- 1 avocado, stone removed, peeled and chopped
- 2 cloves of garlic, chopped
- 2 small red chilli pepper, deseeded
- 1 red pepper (bell pepper), roughly chopped
- 2 tablespoons red wine vinegar
- 2 tablespoons olive oil
- A handful of fresh coriander (cilantro), chopped

SERVES 2

344
calories
per serving

Method

Place the red pepper (bell pepper), chopped garlic, vinegar, oil and chilli into a blender and blitz until smooth. Transfer the mixture to a bowl and add the prawns. Allow them to marinate for at least 30 minutes. Heat a frying pan, add the prawns (shrimps) and cook them for around 5 minutes, or until they are pink and cooked through. Scatter the lettuce leaves on a plate and add the coriander (cilantro) tomato and avocado. Spoon the prawns and the sauce over the top. Serve and enjoy.

Feta & Spinach Slice

Ingredients

225g (8oz) feta cheese, grated (shredded)

125g (4oz) ground almonds

25g (1oz) fresh spinach leaves, chopped

2 eggs

1 onion, finely chopped

1 teaspoon baking powder

200mls (7fl oz) almond milk

**SERVES
3**

378
calories
per serving

Method

Place the spinach into a saucepan, cover it with warm water, bring it to the boil and cook for 3 minutes. Drain it and set aside. Place the ground almonds in a bowl and add in the eggs, milk and baking powder and mix well. Add in the chopped onion, spinach and feta and combine the mixture. Spoon the mixture into a small ovenproof dish and smooth it out. Transfer it to the oven and bake at 190C/375F for 35 minutes. Cut into slices before serving.

Herby Tomato, Cannellini & Feta Salad

Ingredients

400g (14oz) tinned cannellini beans, drained

250g (9oz) cherry tomatoes, halved

75g (3oz) feta cheese, crumbled or diced

50g (2oz) fresh rocket (arugula) leaves

2 tablespoons fresh basil leaves, chopped

1 tablespoon fresh parsley, chopped

2 tablespoons olive oil

Juice of ½ lemon

Sea salt

Freshly ground black pepper

SERVES 2

364
calories
per serving

Method

Place all of the ingredients into a bowl and mix well. Season with salt and pepper. Chill before serving.

Mozzarella & Aubergine Rolls

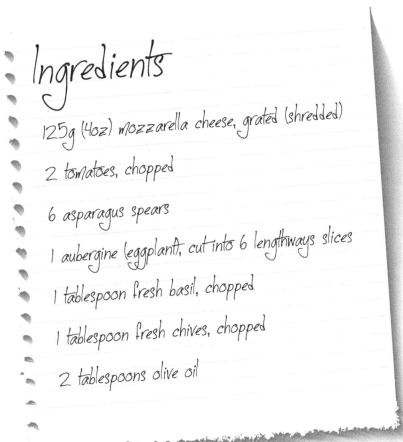

Ingredients

125g (4oz) mozzarella cheese, grated (shredded)

2 tomatoes, chopped

6 asparagus spears

1 aubergine (eggplant, cut into 6 lengthways slices

1 tablespoon fresh basil, chopped

1 tablespoon fresh chives, chopped

2 tablespoons olive oil

SERVES 2

336
calories
per serving

Method

Heat the olive oil in a frying pan, add in the aubergine (eggplant) slices and cook for 2-3 minutes on each side. In the meantime, steam the asparagus for 5 minutes until it has softened. Place the aubergine slices onto plates and sprinkle some cheese, tomatoes and herbs onto each slice. Add an asparagus spear. Roll the aubergine slices up and secure it with a cocktail stick. Serve and enjoy.

Prawn & Cannellini Avocados

Ingredients

300g (11oz) tinned cannellini beans, drained
300g (11oz) cooked, shelled prawns (shrimps)
2 avocados, halved with stone removed
1 red pepper (bell pepper), finely chopped
2 cloves of garlic, crushed
1 tablespoon fresh coriander (cilantro)
½ teaspoon ground paprika
2 tablespoons olive oil
Juice of ½ lemon
Sea salt
Freshly ground black pepper

SERVES 4

333 calories per serving

Method

Pour the lemon juice and olive oil into a bowl and mix well. Stir in the cannellini beans, prawns (shrimps) red pepper (bell pepper), coriander (cilantro), garlic, paprika, salt and black pepper. Mix together until the ingredients are coated with the dressing. Serve the avocado halves onto plates and scoop the prawn mixture on top.

Pancetta & Kidney Bean Salad

Ingredients

400g (14oz) tin of cooked kidney beans,
100g (3½ oz) pancetta, diced
1 red pepper (bell pepper), finely chopped
3 tablespoons red wine vinegar
2 tablespoons fresh chives, chopped
1 tablespoon fresh basil, chopped
1 tablespoon olive oil
1 teaspoon smooth mustard
Sea salt
Freshly ground black pepper

SERVES 2

358
calories
per serving

Method

Heat a frying pan, add the pancetta and cook until crispy. Remove it and set it aside to cool. In a bowl, mix together the oil, vinegar, chives, basil and mustard. Stir in the red pepper (bell pepper), kidney beans and pancetta. Season with salt and pepper. Chill before serving.

Italian Lentil Salad

Ingredients

450g (1lb) green lentils

100g (3½ oz) hazelnuts, chopped

2 spring onions (scallions), chopped

1 cucumber, peeled and diced

1 red pepper (bell pepper), sliced

1 handful of fresh basil

Zest and juice of 1 lemon

100mls (3½ fl oz) olive oil

Sea salt

Freshly ground black pepper

**SERVES
4**

362
calories
per serving

Method

Cook the lentils according to the instructions then allow them to cool. Pour the olive oil and lemon juice into a jug and combine them. Season with salt and pepper. Place all the ingredients for the salad into a bowl and pour on the olive oil and lemon juice.

Avocado & Beetroot Salad

Ingredients

3 small cooked beetroots, sliced

1 small avocado, stone removed, peeled and sliced

1 handful of fresh spinach leaves

2 teaspoons olive oil

1/2 teaspoon paprika

1 teaspoon lemon juice

Sea salt

Freshly ground black pepper

SERVES 1

341 calories per serving

Method

Scatter the spinach leaves on to a plate. Lay the slices of beetroot and avocado on top of the leaves. In a small bowl, mix together the oil, paprika and lemon juice. Season with salt and pepper. Pour the oil dressing over the salad. Enjoy straight away.

Greek Style Salad

Ingredients

350g (12oz) tomatoes, chopped
150g (5oz) feta cheese, crumbled
50g (2oz) pitted black olives, chopped
1 small onion, peeled and chopped
1 iceberg lettuce, finely chopped
1 cucumber, de-seeded and chopped
DRESSING:
3 tablespoons olive oil
Juice of 1 lemon
Sea salt
Freshly ground black pepper

**SERVES
4**

371
calories
per serving

Method

In a bowl, mix together the dressing ingredients. Place all of the salad ingredients into a bowl and add in the dressing. Toss the salad well before serving.

Chicken Lasagne

Ingredients

450g (1lb) chicken either minced (ground) or finely diced

350g (12oz) ricotta cheese

250g (9oz) mozzarella cheese, grated (shredded)

2 x 400g (14oz) tins of chopped tomatoes

4 courgettes (zucchinis) sliced lengthways

3 tablespoons fresh basil, chopped

3 garlic cloves, peeled and chopped

1 onion, chopped

2 red peppers (bell peppers), chopped

1 teaspoon dried oregano

1 teaspoon dried mixed herbs

1 egg

2 teaspoons olive oil

Sea salt

SERVES 6

398 calories per serving

Method

Grease a baking sheet and lay the courgette (zucchini) slices on it. Season with salt, transfer it to the oven and bake at 190C/375F for 15 minutes. In the meantime, heat the oil in a saucepan, add the onions, garlic and red pepper (bell pepper) and cook for 5 minutes. Add in the chicken and cook for 4 minutes. Stir in the tomatoes, basil and oregano and mixed herbs. Bring it to the boil, reduce the heat and simmer for 30 minutes. In a bowl combine the egg and ricotta cheese then set aside. When the chicken mixture is cooked, spoon half of it into an ovenproof dish. Add a layer of the baked courgettes then spoon on half of the ricotta mixture and a layer of mozzarella, repeat with the remaining mixture. Transfer it to the oven and bake at 375F/180C for 40 minutes. Serve with a leafy green salad.

Lemon & Herb Lamb Chops

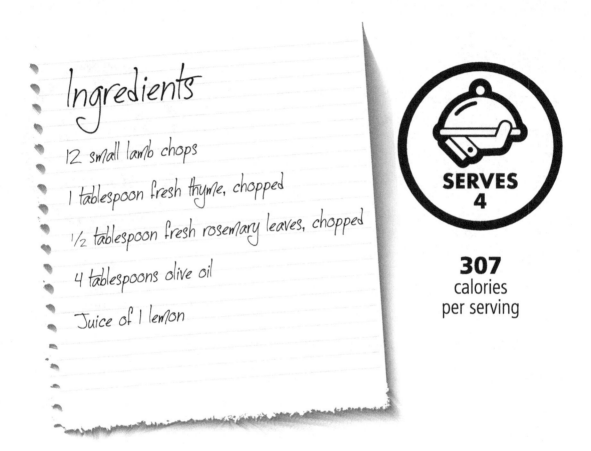

Ingredients

12 small lamb chops

1 tablespoon fresh thyme, chopped

½ tablespoon fresh rosemary leaves, chopped

4 tablespoons olive oil

Juice of 1 lemon

SERVES 4

307 calories per serving

Method

Pour the oil into a bowl and stir in the lemon juice, rosemary and thyme. Place the lamb chops in the mixture and allow it to marinate for at least 1 hour or overnight if you can. Transfer the chops to a hot grill (broiler) and cook for 5 minutes on either side or until the chops are cooked to your liking. Serve with a heap of salad or roast vegetables.

Salmon, Butter Beans & Yogurt Dressing

Ingredients

400g (14oz) butter beans
125g (4oz) plain Greek yogurt
4 salmon fillets
3 cloves of garlic, chopped
1 red chilli, finely chopped
½ teaspoon paprika, plus extra for seasoning
½ teaspoon oregano
1 tablespoon olive oil
Zest and juice ½ lemon
Sea salt
Freshly ground black pepper

SERVES 4

385 calories per serving

Method

Place the yogurt into a bowl and add in the lemon juice and paprika. Heat the oil in a pan, add the oregano, garlic and chilli and warm them for 2 minutes. Add in the butter beans and lemon zest and warm them through. Sprinkle the paprika over the salmon and season it with salt and pepper. Place the salmon fillets under a hot grill (broiler) and cook for around 8 minutes, or until completely cooked, turning half way through. Serve the salmon with the butter beans and a dollop of yogurt dressing.

Hunters Chicken

Ingredients

- 400g (14oz) broccoli florets
- 250g (8oz) tomato passata
- 75g (3½ oz) mozzarella cheese, grated (shredded)
- 4 slices of bacon
- 4 chicken breasts
- 1 onion, chopped
- 2 teaspoons olive oil

SERVES 4

394 calories per serving

Method

Heat the oil in a frying pan, add the onion and cook for 5 minutes. Add the passata and cook for 10 minutes to reduce the mixture. Place the chicken flat-side down on a lightly greased ovenproof dish and make an incision to make room for the sauce. Spoon the sauce into the incision. Wrap a slice of bacon around each chicken breast. Transfer the chicken to the oven and cook for 25 minutes. Scatter the cheese over the chicken breasts and return them to the oven for 5 minutes or until the cheese is bubbling. In the mean-time steam or boil the broccoli for 5 minutes. Serve the broccoli onto plates and add the chicken.

Spiced Chicken & Courgette Salad

Ingredients

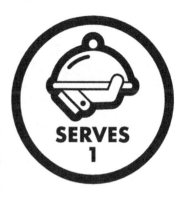

SERVES 1

314 calories per serving

25g (1oz) chargrilled artichokes in oil, drained and chopped

1 chicken breast, cut into strips

1 medium courgettes (zucchini), sliced lengthways

1 handful of rocket (arugula) leaves

1 teaspoon olive oil

1 teaspoon balsamic vinegar

½ teaspoon harissa paste

Method

Place the harissa paste and olive oil in a bowl and coat the chicken in the mixture. Heat a griddle pan on a high heat and lay the courgette (zucchini) slices on it. Cook them until they have softened slightly then set them aside and keep warm. Place the chicken in the pan and cook it for around 6 minutes or until cooked completely, turning it over halfway through. Scatter the rocket (arugula) leaves onto a plate together with the artichoke pieces. Add the courgette and chicken to the salad. Drizzle the balsamic vinegar over the top. Serve and eat straight away.

Rack of Lamb With Cucumber & Hummus

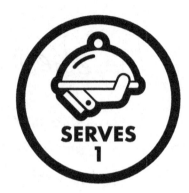

SERVES 1

354 calories per serving

Ingredients

- 5cm (2 inch) chunk of cucumber, sliced
- 1 tablespoon hummus
- 1 rack of lamb (3 cutlets)
- 2 teaspoons olive oil
- 1/2 teaspoon ground cumin
- 1/2 teaspoon ground coriander (cilantro)
- 1/2 teaspoon all-spice

Method

Place the oil, cumin, coriander (cilantro) and all-spice into a bowl and mix well. Coat the lamb in the mixture. Place the lamb in a roasting tin and cook in the oven at 220C/445F for 15-20 minutes or until the lamb has browned. Place the cucumber onto a plate and add a dollop of hummus and serve the lamb. Enjoy straight away.

Mustard & Garlic Prawns

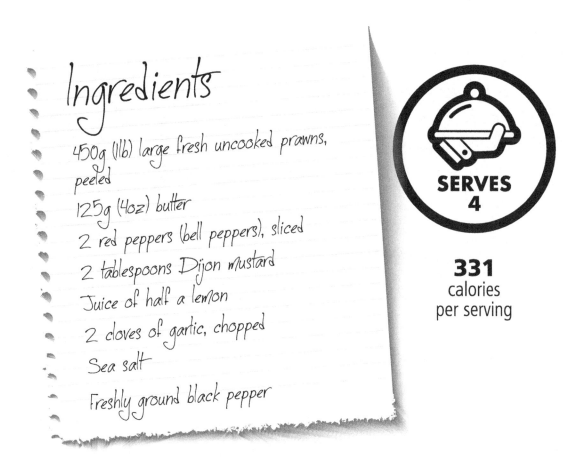

Ingredients

450g (1lb) large fresh uncooked prawns, peeled

125g (4oz) butter

2 red peppers (bell peppers), sliced

2 tablespoons Dijon mustard

Juice of half a lemon

2 cloves of garlic, chopped

Sea salt

Freshly ground black pepper

SERVES 4

331 calories per serving

Method

Place the prawns in an ovenproof dish and scatter the red peppers (bell peppers) into the dish. Heat the butter in a small saucepan and stir in the mustard, garlic and lemon juice. Warm the mixture until the butter has melted. Pour the butter over the prawns and peppers. Season with salt and pepper. Transfer to the oven and bake at 220C/425F for 15 minutes or until the prawns are pink and completely cooked.

Marinated Pork Chops

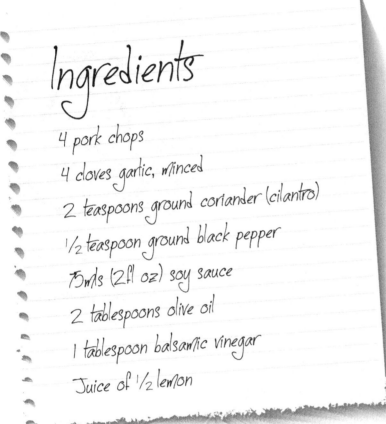

Ingredients

- 4 pork chops
- 4 cloves garlic, minced
- 2 teaspoons ground coriander (cilantro)
- ½ teaspoon ground black pepper
- 75mls (2fl oz) soy sauce
- 2 tablespoons olive oil
- 1 tablespoon balsamic vinegar
- Juice of ½ lemon

**SERVES
4**

320
calories
per serving

Method

Place the garlic, balsamic, soy sauce, lemon juice, olive oil, coriander (cilantro) and pepper in a bowl and mix well. Add the pork chops to the bowl and coat them thoroughly in the mixture. Cover and refrigerate them for at least 30 minutes, or overnight if you can. When they are sufficiently marinated, heat a frying pan and add the chops together with all of the marinade. Cook for 5 minutes on each side, or until the chops are thoroughly cooked. Serve with a heap of green salad and cauliflower rice.

Tomato, Feta & Pomegranate Bake

Ingredients

450g (1lb) cherry tomatoes, halved

75g (3oz) pomegranate seeds

2 blocks of feta cheese, halved widthways

2 teaspoons ground coriander

½ teaspoon chilli powder

1 tablespoon olive oil

1 handful of fresh parsley, chopped

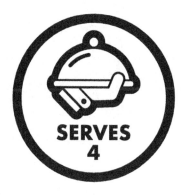

SERVES 4

328 calories per serving

Method

Scatter the tomatoes into an oven proof dish, and sprinkle with coriander (cilantro) and chilli powder. Transfer it to the oven and cook at 220C/440F for 15 minutes. Lay the feta on top of the tomato mixture, drizzle with the olive oil. Return it to the oven and continue cooking for 7-10 minutes or until the feta is golden. Sprinkle with the pomegranate seeds and parsley. Serve with a heap of green salad.

Salmon Kebabs

Ingredients

8 button mushrooms

8 pitted black olives

4 salmon fillets

2 tablespoons fresh parsley, chopped

Juice and rind of 1 lemon

3 tablespoons olive oil

**SERVES
4**

385
calories
per serving

Method

Cut the salmon into chunks and place them in a bowl. Squeeze in the lemon juice and add the rind, olive oil and parsley and coat the salmon chunks thoroughly. Add the mushrooms and coat them in the dressing too. Thread the fish, olives and mushrooms onto skewers. Place them under a hot grill (broiler) and cook for 4-5 minutes turning occasionally.

Spicy Meatballs & Minty Yogurt Dip

Ingredients

450g (1lb) minced turkey (or beef)

50g (2oz) ground almonds

3 tablespoons harissa paste

1 tablespoon tomato purée (paste)

2 garlic cloves, crushed

Juice of 1 lemon

1 egg

2 tablespoons olive oil

FOR THE DIP:
200g (7oz) plain yogurt (unflavoured)

12 mint leaves, finely chopped

SERVES 4

346 calories per serving

Method

In a bowl, combine the turkey with 2 tablespoons of harissa paste, the almonds, garlic, lemon juice and egg and mix really well. Scoop portions of the mixture out with a spoon and shape into balls. Cover and refrigerate for 40 minutes. Heat the oil in a frying pan, add a tablespoon of harissa paste and tomato purée (paste) and stir. Add the meatballs and cook for 7-8 minutes, turning occasionally until thoroughly cooked. In the meantime, combine the yogurt and mint and mix well. Skewer each meatball with a cocktail stick and serve ready to be dipped in the yogurt. Enjoy.

Halloumi & Vegetable Traybake

SERVES 4

378
calories
per serving

Ingredients

- 350g (1lb) halloumi cheese, thickly sliced
- 25g (1oz) pine nuts
- 8 cherry tomatoes, halved
- 3 cloves of garlic, chopped
- 2 onions, peeled and chopped
- 1 yellow pepper (bell pepper), deseeded and chopped
- 1 red pepper (bell pepper), deseeded and chopped
- 1 handful of fresh basil, chopped
- 1 handful of fresh parsley, chopped
- 1 tablespoon olive oil
- 2 teaspoons paprika

Method

Preheat the oven to 200C/400F. Scatter the tomatoes, onions, peppers and garlic into a roasting tin. Coat them in paprika and olive oil. Toss them well in the mixture. Lay the halloumi on top of the vegetables. Transfer it to the oven and cook for 25 minutes or until the halloumi is golden. Add in the parsley, basil and pine nuts and serve.

Recipes Under 500 Calories

Pork Steaks, Peppers & Beans

Ingredients

- 400g (14oz) cannellini beans, drained
- 8 pork steaks
- 4 tablespoons fresh parsley, chopped
- 2 red peppers (bell peppers)
- 1 onion, chopped
- 1 tablespoon red wine vinegar
- 1 tablespoon olive oil
- Sea salt
- Freshly ground black pepper

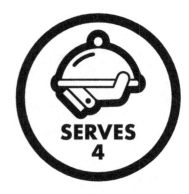

SERVES 4

460 calories per serving

Method

Season the pork steaks with salt and pepper. Heat the olive oil in a frying pan, add the pork and cook for around 3 minutes on each side. Remove them, set aside and keep them warm. Add the peppers (bell peppers) and onion to the pan and cook for 5 minutes until the vegetables have softened. Add the parsley, vinegar and beans and warm them thoroughly. Serve the pork steaks and spoon the vegetables over the top. Enjoy.

Tuna & Lentil Bake

Ingredients

200g (7oz) tinned tuna in brine, drained

250g (9oz) lentils

50g (2oz) cheese, grated (shredded)

1 onion, peeled and finely chopped

1 carrot, peeled and finely chopped

1 handful of fresh parsley, chopped

1 handful of fresh chives, chopped

450mls (15fl oz) vegetable stock (broth)

1 tablespoon olive oil

SERVES 4

448 calories per serving

Method

Preheat the oven to 200C/400F. Pour the stock (broth) into a saucepan, add the lentils and cook for 12 minutes. Drizzle the olive oil into an ovenproof dish. Scatter the lentils into the dish and add the flaked tuna, onion, carrot and herbs and mix well. Sprinkle the cheese over the top. Transfer it to the oven and cook for around 20 minutes. Serve and eat straight away.

Avocado & Chicken Omelette

Ingredients

- 25g (1oz) cheese, grated (shredded)
- 50g (2oz) leftover chicken, chopped
- 2 eggs, beaten
- Flesh of ½ avocado, chopped
- 1 teaspoon fresh basil
- 1 teaspoon olive oil
- Freshly ground black pepper

SERVES 1

491 calories per serving

Method

Heat the olive oil in a frying pan then pour in the beaten egg. While it begins to set sprinkle on the grated cheese, basil, chicken and chopped avocado. Cook until the eggs are completely set and the cheese has melted. Season with black pepper.

Salmon & Olive Bake

Ingredients

450g (1lb) courgettes (zucchinis), roughly chopped

2 x 400g (2x14oz) tinned chopped tomatoes

100g (3½ oz) black olives in brine, drained

4 salmon fillets

1 onion, roughly chopped

2 tablespoons fresh basil

2 tablespoons fresh parsley

1 tablespoon olive oil

**SERVES
4**

453
calories
per serving

Method

Preheat the oven to 200C/400F. Add the olive oil, onion, courgette (zucchini), tinned tomatoes, olives, basil and parsley to the roasting tin and cook in the oven for 10 minutes. Lay the salmon fillets on top. Return the roasting tin to the oven and cook for 12-15 minutes or until the salmon is completely cooked. Serve and enjoy!

Desserts Under 230 Calories

Spiced Poached Pears

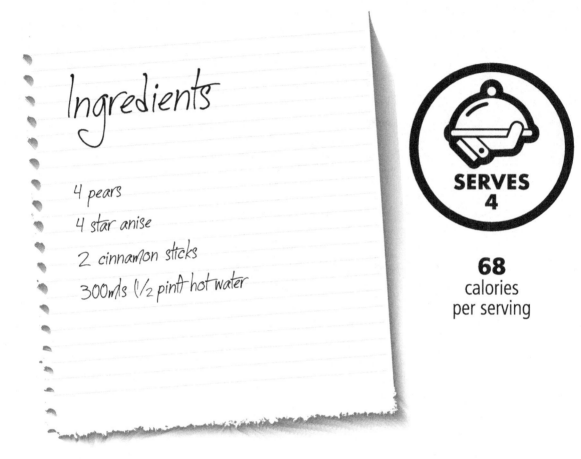

Ingredients

4 pears

4 star anise

2 cinnamon sticks

300mls (½ pint) hot water

SERVES 4

68
calories
per serving

Method

Place the water, star anise and cinnamon into a saucepan and bring it to the boil. Add the pears, reduce the heat and simmer gently for 10 minutes. Remove them from the water and serve.

Chocolate Truffles

Ingredients

- 75g (3oz) smooth peanut butter
- 50g (2oz) desiccated (shredded) coconut
- 25g (1oz) chia seeds
- 25g (1oz) coconut oil
- 2 teaspoons coconut flour
- 1 tablespoon 100% cocoa powder
- 1 tablespoon stevia sweetener
- Cocoa powder for coating (approx. 1 tablespoon)

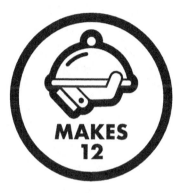

MAKES 12

102 calories per ball

Method

Place all the ingredients into a bowl or food processor (apart from the cocoa powder for coating) and process until smooth. Using a teaspoon, scoop out a little of the mixture, shape it into a ball and roll it in cocoa powder. Chill before serving.

Nutty Chocolate Treats

Ingredients

125g (4oz) walnuts, chopped

125g (4oz) almonds, chopped

50g (2oz) coconut oil

50g (2oz) desiccated (shredded) coconut

2 eggs, beaten

2 tablespoons peanut butter

2 tablespoons 100% cocoa powder (or cacao nibs)

2 tablespoons tahini (sesame) paste

1 tablespoon sunflower seeds

1 tablespoon stevia

1 teaspoon ground cinnamon

1 handful of fresh chives, chopped

450mls (15fl oz) vegetable stock (broth)

1 tablespoon olive oil

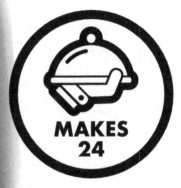

MAKES 24

128 calories per serving

Method

Place all the ingredients into a bowl or a food processor and mix it well, keeping the nuts a nice chunky texture. Spoon the mixture into small paper baking cases. Transfer them to the oven and bake at 180C/360F for 20 minutes. Allow them to cool then store them in an airtight container.

Berry Compote & Vanilla Yogurt

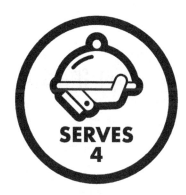

SERVES 4

139 calories per serving

Ingredients

250g (9oz) blueberries

250g (9oz) strawberries

100g (3½ oz) redcurrants

100g (3½ oz) blackberries

4 tablespoons plain yogurt

½ teaspoon vanilla essence

Zest and juice of 1 orange

Method

Place all of the berries into a pan along with the orange zest and juice. Gently heat the berries for around 5 minutes until warmed through. Mix the vanilla essence into the yogurt. Serve the berries with a dollop of yogurt on top.

Tropical Skewers & Fruit Sauce

SERVES 4

167
calories
per serving

Ingredients

2 bananas, peeled and thickly sliced

1 pineapple, (approx. 2lb weight) peeled and diced

400g (14oz) strawberries

1 teaspoon 100% cocoa powder or cacao nibs

Method

Place the cocoa powder/cacao nibs and 125g (4oz) of strawberries into a food processor and blitz until creamy. Pour the sauce into a serving bowl. Skewer the bananas, pineapple chunks and remaining strawberries onto skewers. Serve the sauce alongside the skewers.

Raspberry Cupcakes

Ingredients

250g (9oz) ground almonds (almond flour/almond meal)

150g (5oz) fresh raspberries

3 eggs, whisked

1 teaspoon baking powder

1 teaspoon stevia powder (or to taste)

50mls (2fl oz) melted coconut oil

Pinch of salt

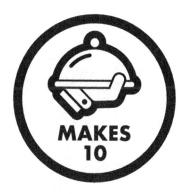

MAKES 10

228 calories each

Method

Lightly grease a 10-hole muffin tin. In a bowl, combine the ground almonds (almond flour/almond meal), baking powder, stevia and salt. In another bowl, combine the coconut oil and eggs then pour the mixture into the dry ingredients. Mix well. Add the raspberries to the mixture and gently stir them in. Spoon some of the mixture into each of the muffin moulds. Transfer them to the oven and bake at 170C/325F for around 20 minutes or until golden.

You may also be interested in other titles by
Erin Rose Publishing
which are available in both paperback and ebook.

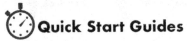 Quick Start Guides

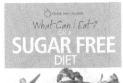
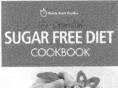
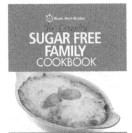
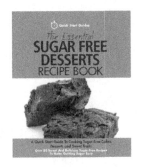
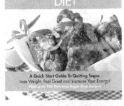
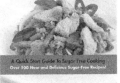

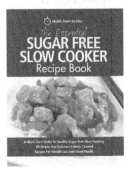
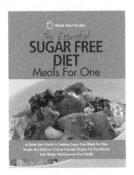
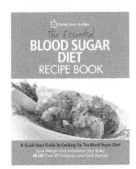
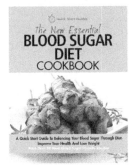

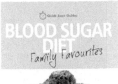
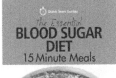
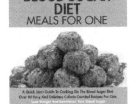
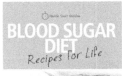
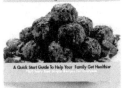
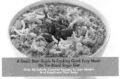
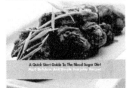

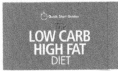
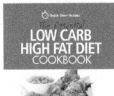
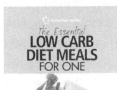
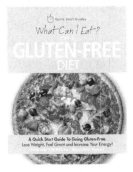
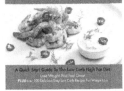
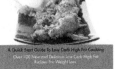
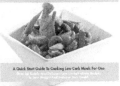

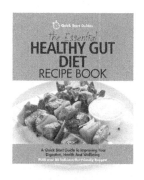

Quick Start Guides

The Essential
HEALTHY GUT DIET
RECIPE BOOK

A Quick Start Guide To Improving Your
Digestion, Health And Wellbeing
PLUS over 80 Delicious Gut-Friendly Recipes

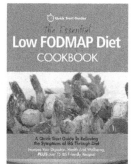

Quick Start Guides

The Essential
Low FODMAP Diet
COOKBOOK

A Quick Start Guide To Relieving
the Symptoms of IBS Through Diet
Improve Your Digestion, Health And Wellbeing
PLUS over 75 IBS Friendly Recipes

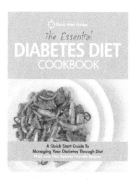

Quick Start Guides

The Essential
DIABETES DIET
COOKBOOK

A Quick Start Guide To
Managing Your Diabetes Through Diet

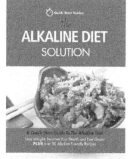

Quick Start Guides

The
ALKALINE DIET
SOLUTION

A Quick Start Guide To The Alkaline Diet
Lose Weight, Increase Your Health and Feel Great
PLUS over 90 Alkaline-Friendly Recipes

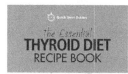

Quick Start Guides

The Essential
THYROID DIET
RECIPE BOOK

A Quick Start Guide To Healing Your Thyroid
Through Diet, Lose Weight And Feel Great
With Delicious Thyroid Friendly Recipes

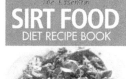

Quick Start Guides

The Essential
SIRT FOOD
DIET RECIPE BOOK

A Quick Start Guide to Cooking on the SIRT Food Diet
Over 100 Easy and Delicious Recipes to Burn Fat,
Lose Weight, Get Lean and Feel Great!

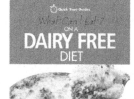

Quick Start Guides

What Can I Eat?
ON A
DAIRY FREE
DIET

A Quick Start Guide To Quitting Dairy and Lactose
Lose Weight, Feel Great and Increase Your Energy
PLUS 100 Delicious Dairy-Free Recipes

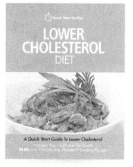

Quick Start Guides

The
LOWER
CHOLESTEROL
DIET

A Quick Start Guide To Lower Cholesterol
Improve Your Health and Feel Great
PLUS over 100 Delicious Cholesterol-Lowering Recipes

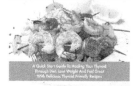

Quick Start Guides

THE VEGAN
15 MINUTE
COOKBOOK

Over 100 Simple And Delicious
Vegan Recipes For Everyone

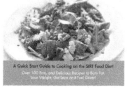

Quick Start Guides

The Essential
ROASTING TIN
COOKBOOK

Over 80 Easy And Delicious
One Dish, No-Fuss Oven Recipes

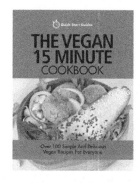

Blood Sugar Diet
Diary

Daily Diary To Track Health, Weight Loss
And Wellbeing On the Blood Sugar Diet

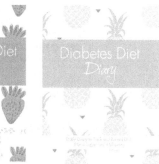

Diabetes Diet
Diary

Daily Diary to Track and Control Diet
The Sugar and Wellbeing

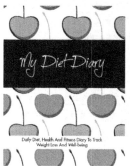

My Diet Diary

Daily Diet, Health And Fitness Diary To Track
Weight Loss And Well-being

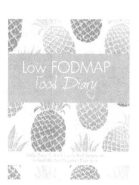

Low FODMAP
Food Diary

Daily Diary To Track Foods And Symptoms
To Beat IBS And Digestive Disorders

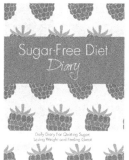

Sugar-Free Diet
Diary

Daily Diary For Quitting Sugar,
Losing Weight and Feeling Great

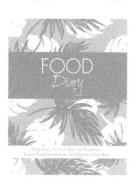

FOOD
Diary

Daily Diary To Track Diet And Symptoms
To Beat Food Intolerances And Digestive Disorders

You may also be interested in titles by
Pomegranate Journals

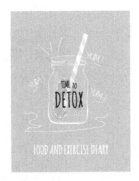
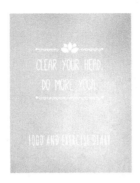
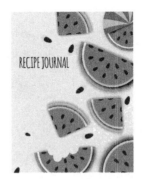
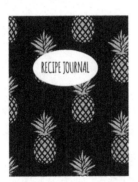
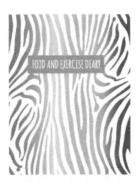
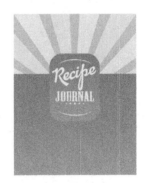
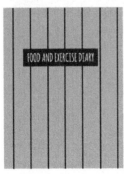

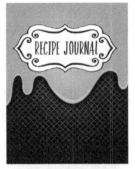
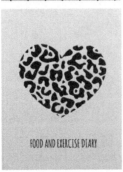
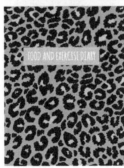
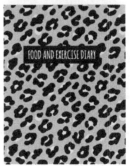

Made in the USA
Coppell, TX
13 July 2020